6 MINUTE FITNESS AT 50+

CORE EXERCISES FOR BALANCE AND STRENGTH

GARY A. PRY

COPYRIGHT

Copyright © 2023 by Gary A. Pry

OTHER BOOKS BY AUTHOR

GREEN SMOOTHIE RECIPES FOR SENIORS

PEGAN DIET COOKBOOK FOR NOVICE

PLANT BASED JUICING RECIPES

(GET ACCESS TO IT IN THE KINDLE VERSION OF THIS BOOK)

TABLE OF CONTENT

INTRODUCTION

At 50, Martha stumbled upon an old fitness book while cleaning out her attic. Curiosity piqued, she dusted it off and started reading. It was a treasure trove of exercise routines and healthy living tips specifically designed for seniors.

Eager to reclaim her vitality, Martha followed the book religiously. Step by step, she adopted a well-rounded fitness routine, including gentle exercises, yoga, and balanced nutrition. Gradually, she felt her strength and flexibility improve.

But the book offered more than just physical guidance. It became her companion, motivating her through challenging days. Martha's newfound energy extended to her social life too, as she joined a local seniors' fitness class. Surrounded by like-minded individuals, she formed lasting friendships.

With each passing day, Martha's zest for life grew, proving that age was never a barrier to transformation. The book 6 MINUTE FITNESS AT 50 had breathed new life into her golden years, reminding her that the pursuit of wellness is timeless and rewarding.

CHAPTER ONE

PHYSICAL FITNESS

Physical fitness refers to the state of being physically healthy, strong, and capable of performing daily activities with ease. It involves a combination of cardiovascular endurance, muscular strength and endurance, flexibility, and body composition.

TYPES OF EXERCISE FOR SENIORS

Cardiovascular (Aerobic) Exercise: Activities like walking, swimming, cycling, and dancing help improve cardiovascular health, strengthen the heart, and enhance lung capacity. Cardio exercises also aid in managing weight, reducing the risk of heart disease, and boosting energy levels.

Strength Training: It involves using resistance, for example resistance bands to build muscle strength. Strength training helps maintain muscle mass, bone density, and joint health, reducing the risk of falls and fractures. It also improves metabolism and overall physical function.

Flexibility Exercises: Stretching exercises enhance flexibility, mobility, and balance. They can help alleviate joint stiffness, reduce the risk of injuries, and improve posture.

Balance Exercises: Balance training is essential for older adults to prevent falls and maintain stability. Activities like tai chi and yoga can improve balance and coordination.

Low-Impact Exercises: Low-impact activities like water aerobics or elliptical training are gentle on joints, making them ideal for seniors with joint issues or arthritis.

Mind-Body Exercises: Mind-body practices like yoga and meditation can help reduce stress, improve mental clarity, and promote relaxation and overall well-being.

THE IMPORTANCE OF EXERCISE FOR SENIORS

Improved Cognitive Function: Regular exercise has been linked to better cognitive function and a reduced risk of cognitive decline and dementia.

Mood Enhancement: Exercise can positively impact mental health, reducing the risk of depression and anxiety while promoting a sense of well-being.

Social Interaction: Group exercises offer opportunities for social engagement and combat feelings of isolation.

Maintaining Independence: By improving strength, flexibility, and balance, exercise helps seniors maintain their independence and perform daily activities more easily.

Chronic Disease Management: Regular physical activity can help manage various chronic conditions like diabetes, hypertension, and arthritis, leading to better overall health outcomes.

MYTHS OF SENIORS EXERCISING

1. **Myth: Seniors should avoid exercise to prevent injuries.**

    - Fact: While it's true that seniors need to be cautious and mindful of their bodies, regular exercise can actually help prevent injuries by improving strength, balance, and flexibility.

2. **Myth: Exercise is only for younger people, not for seniors.**

    - Fact: Exercise is beneficial for people of all ages, including seniors. Age is not a barrier to starting or continuing a fitness routine.

3. **Myth: Seniors are too old to build muscle or gain strength.**

    - Fact: Seniors can build muscle and gain strength through strength training exercises. While the rate of muscle gain may be slower than in younger individuals, it is still achievable.

4. **Myth: Cardio exercises are too strenuous for seniors.**

    - Fact: Low-impact cardio exercises, such as walking, swimming, or cycling, are generally safe and beneficial for seniors' cardiovascular health.

5. **Myth: Seniors should avoid weightlifting as it may lead to joint problems.**

   - Fact: When performed with proper form and appropriate weight, weightlifting can be safe and beneficial for seniors. It can help maintain bone density and strengthen muscles around the joints, reducing the risk of joint problems.

6. **Myth: Seniors should rest and avoid physical activity to conserve energy.**

   - Fact: Inactivity can lead to muscle weakness and decreased energy levels. Regular physical activity actually helps maintain energy levels and overall vitality.

7. **Myth: Seniors with chronic health conditions should avoid exercise.**

   - Fact: In many cases, exercise can be beneficial for seniors with chronic conditions. However, it's important to consult with a healthcare provider to determine the most suitable exercise plan.

8. **Myth: Exercise won't have any impact on cognitive function in seniors.**

   - Fact: Regular exercise has been shown to improve cognitive function and memory in older adults.

9. **Myth: Stretching is not necessary for seniors, as flexibility naturally declines with age.**

- Fact: Stretching is important for seniors to maintain flexibility, improve mobility, and reduce the risk of injuries.

10. **Myth: Seniors should stick to exercises they have always done and avoid trying new activities.**

   - Fact: Seniors can benefit from trying new exercises or activities that suit their interests and physical capabilities, as it keeps the routine enjoyable and engaging.

CHAPTER 2

WHERE TO OBSERVE EXERCISES

Fitness Centers/Gyms: Many fitness centers and gyms offer specialized exercise classes and equipment tailored to seniors' needs. These classes are designed to be low-impact, focusing on strength, balance, flexibility, and cardiovascular health. Seniors can work with fitness trainers who understand their unique requirements and can guide them through appropriate exercises.

Senior Centers: Community centers and senior facilities often provide exercise programs and classes suitable for older adults. These classes may include chair exercises, yoga, tai chi, and low-impact aerobics. Participating in such programs at a senior center can be a great way for older individuals to socialize with peers while staying physically active.

Community Parks: Many community parks have walking paths or outdoor fitness equipment. Walking is an excellent low-impact exercise for seniors, and outdoor fitness equipment provides opportunities for strength and flexibility training in a pleasant environment.

Swimming Pools: Water-based exercises, such as water aerobics or swimming, are particularly beneficial for seniors. The buoyancy of water reduces impact on joints, making it an ideal choice for those with arthritis or joint pain. Swimming and water aerobics provide an effective full-body workout.

Home Workouts: Seniors can exercise in the comfort of their homes using bodyweight exercises, resistance bands, or light dumbbells. There are numerous workout routines available online or through fitness DVDs specifically designed for older adults. Home workouts offer convenience and flexibility for those who prefer exercising at their own pace.

Online Classes: The internet offers a wealth of resources, including online exercise classes and instructional videos specifically tailored to seniors. Virtual classes allow seniors to participate in guided workouts from the comfort of their homes, providing flexibility and accessibility.

MISTAKES TO AVOID DURING EXERCISE:

Overexertion: Seniors should start their exercise routine gradually, especially if they are new to physical activity or haven't been active for a while. Pushing too hard or doing too much too soon can lead to injuries or burnout.

Ignoring Pain: Pain during exercise is a sign that something may be wrong. Seniors should never ignore pain or discomfort and should stop the activity if they experience any unusual sensations. If pain persists, they should consult a healthcare professional.

Not Warming Up: Warming up before exercise is essential to prepare the body for physical activity. A proper warm-up increases blood flow to muscles, improves flexibility, and reduces the risk of injury.

Forgetting to Hydrate: Proper hydration is essential during exercise, as seniors may be more susceptible to dehydration. Drinking water before, during, and after workouts helps maintain energy levels and supports overall health.

Not Balancing Exercises: A well-rounded fitness routine should include a mix of cardio, strength training, flexibility, and balance exercises. Focusing solely on one type of exercise may lead to imbalances and neglect certain areas of fitness.

Skipping Recovery Days: Seniors need sufficient rest and recovery between exercise sessions, especially if they engage in more intense workouts. Rest allows muscles to repair and prevents overtraining, which can lead to fatigue and increased risk of injury.

SAFETY CONSIDERATIONS:

Consulting with Healthcare Providers: Before starting a new exercise program, seniors should consult with their healthcare provider, especially if they have any pre-existing health conditions or concerns.

Proper Form and Technique: Performing exercises with proper form is crucial for preventing injuries and maximizing the benefits. Seniors may consider working with a qualified fitness professional to learn correct movements and techniques.

Using Appropriate Equipment: Seniors should use appropriate exercise equipment, such as supportive footwear and stability aids like canes or walkers, to ensure safety during workouts.

Listening to Their Bodies: Seniors should pay attention to their bodies and adjust their exercise routine as needed. If an exercise causes pain or discomfort, they should modify or avoid it and seek guidance from a healthcare professional or fitness expert.

20 FITNESS EXERCISE

March in Place:

- Stand with feet hip-width apart and lift your knees high, alternating legs.

- Pump your arms back and forth as if you are marching.

- Continue this movement for 30 seconds.

Arm Circles:

- Stand with feet shoulder-width apart and extend your arms straight out to the sides.

- Make small circles with your arms, rotating them forward for 15 seconds.

- Then, reverse the direction and rotate them backward for another 15 seconds.

Shoulder Rolls:

- Stand with feet shoulder-width apart and relax your arms by your sides.

- Roll your shoulders forward in a circular motion for 15 seconds.

- Then, roll them backward in a circular motion for another 15 seconds.

Leg Swings (Front to Back):

- Stand next to a sturdy object (e.g., a table or chair) and hold onto it for balance.

- Swing one leg forward and backward in a controlled manner.

- Perform this movement for 15 seconds on one leg, then switch to the other leg for another 15 seconds.

Leg Swings (Side to Side):

- Stand next to a sturdy object and hold onto it for balance.

- Swing one leg side to side in a controlled manner.

- Perform this movement for 15 seconds on one leg, then switch to the other leg for another 15 seconds.

Knee Lifts:

- Stand with feet hip-width apart.

- Lift your knees as high as comfortable, one at a time, while pumping your arms.

- Continue this movement for 30 seconds.

Toe Touches:

- Stand tall with feet shoulder-width apart.

- Reach your arms up toward the ceiling and then bend at the waist to touch your toes.

- Repeat this movement for 30 seconds.

Side Reaches:

- Stand with feet shoulder-width apart.

- Reach one arm up and over your head, bending slightly to the opposite side.

- Return to the starting position and switch to the other side.

- Continue alternating side reaches for 30 seconds.

Heel Raises:

- Stand tall with feet hip-width apart.

- Lift your heels off the ground, rising onto the balls of your feet.

- Lower your heels back down to the ground and repeat for 30 seconds.

Chair Squats:

- Stand in front of a sturdy chair with feet shoulder-width apart.

- Slowly lower yourself into a sitting position on the chair, as if you're about to sit down.

- Just before touching the chair, push through your heels to stand back up.

- Repeat this movement for 30 seconds.

Wall Push-Ups:

- Stand facing a wall with arms extended and palms flat against the wall.

- Slowly bend your elbows and lower your chest toward the wall.

- Push yourself back to the starting position by straightening your arms.

- Repeat this movement for 30 seconds.

Bicep Curls:

- Hold light dumbbells or resistance bands in your hands, palms facing forward.

- Slowly bend your elbows, bringing the weights toward your shoulders.

- Lower the weights back down to the starting position.

- Repeat this movement for 30 seconds.

Tricep Dips:

- Sit on a sturdy chair with your hands gripping the edge of the seat.

- Slide your bottom off the chair, supporting your weight with your arms.

- Bend your elbows to lower yourself toward the floor.

- Push through your palms to raise yourself back up.

- Repeat this movement for 30 seconds.

Seated Leg Extensions:

- Sit on a chair with feet flat on the floor.

- Lift one leg, extending it straight out in front of you.

- Lower the leg back down and switch to the other leg.

- Continue alternating leg extensions for 30 seconds.

Ankle Circles:

- Sit on a chair and lift one foot off the ground.

- Make circles with your ankle in one direction for 15 seconds.

- Then, reverse the direction of the circles for another 15 seconds.

- Switch to the other foot and repeat.

Neck Rotations:

- Sit or stand with a straight back.

- Gently rotate your neck to the left, bringing your chin toward your shoulder.

- Slowly return to the center and then rotate to the right.

- Continue alternating neck rotations for 30 seconds.

Wrist Flexion and Extension:

- Sit or stand with your arms extended in front of you.

- Gently bend your wrists upward, pointing your fingers toward the ceiling.

- Then, bend your wrists downward, pointing your fingers toward the floor.

- Continue alternating wrist flexion and extension for 30 seconds.

Calf Stretches:

- Stand facing a wall, about an arm's length away.

- Step one foot back and press the heel of that foot into the ground.

- Keep your back leg straight and feel the stretch in your calf.

- Hold the stretch for 15 seconds and then switch to the other leg.

Hip Flexor Stretch:

- Stand near a chair or a wall for support.

- Step one foot back, bending the knee slightly and keeping the other leg in front.

- Gently lower your body toward the floor, feeling the stretch in the front of your hip.

- Hold the stretch for 15 seconds and then switch to the other leg.

Deep Breathing:

Sit or stand with a straight back and relax your shoulders.

Inhale deeply through your nose, expanding your lungs.

Exhale slowly through your mouth, releasing all the air.

Continue deep breathing for the last 30 seconds to cool down and relax.

Remember to perform each exercise with control and within your comfort level. If you experience any pain or discomfort during the workout, stop immediately and consult a healthcare professional.

Additionally, warm up before starting the exercises and cool down afterward to prevent injury and enhance flexibility. Enjoy your 7-minute workout for seniors!

FOODS TO EAT

Salmon: High in omega-3 fatty acids, which support joint health and reduce inflammation.

Spinach: Packed with vitamins, minerals, and antioxidants to support overall health.

Greek Yogurt: Rich in protein and calcium, promoting muscle strength and bone health.

Berries (Blueberries, Strawberries, etc.): Loaded with antioxidants that aid in reducing oxidative stress.

Sweet Potatoes: A great source of complex carbohydrates and vitamins for sustained energy.

Quinoa: Contains complete proteins and fiber, supporting muscle repair and digestion.

Nuts (Almonds, Walnuts, etc.): High in healthy fats and protein, helping to keep energy levels steady.

Lean Chicken or Turkey: A good source of protein for muscle maintenance and repair.

Beans and Lentils: High in protein and fiber, contributing to overall health and well-being.

Avocado: Packed with healthy fats and essential nutrients to support heart health.

Oats: Rich in fiber and provide lasting energy for an active lifestyle.

Oranges: High in vitamin C, which aids in collagen formation and supports joint health.

Broccoli: Contains antioxidants and vitamins for overall health and immune support.

Eggs: A complete protein source, important for muscle health and repair.

Tofu: High in protein and a good plant-based alternative for muscle support.

Cottage Cheese: Rich in protein and calcium, beneficial for bone health.

Pumpkin Seeds: Contain magnesium, zinc, and antioxidants for overall well-being.

Whole Grains (Brown Rice, Whole Wheat, etc.): Provide sustained energy and essential nutrients.

Brussels Sprouts: High in vitamin K, supporting bone health and blood clotting.

Cauliflower: A versatile vegetable rich in vitamins and antioxidants for overall health.

These foods are not only nutritious but also versatile, allowing seniors to enjoy them in various dishes and meal plans.

Remember that a balanced diet, along with regular physical activity, is essential for maintaining strength and overall physical fitness as we age. It's always a good idea for seniors to consult with a healthcare professional or a registered dietitian for personalized dietary advice.

CONCLUSION

As we close the chapters of this book, we find ourselves inspired by the remarkable resilience and determination of our seniors. 6 MINUTES FITNESS AT 5O has been a testament to the transformative power of exercise in the golden years. From dispelling myths to outlining the significance of daily physical activity, we have unraveled the true potential that lies within each senior.

Together, we explored the diverse places where seniors can embrace their exercise journey, fostering a sense of community and camaraderie along the way. From bustling gyms to serene community parks, from the inviting waters of swimming pools to the comfort of home, the world has become a boundless playground for our esteemed seniors.

Recognizing that physical fitness knows no age, we have unveiled the importance of exercise for seniors, not merely as a means to maintain strength but as an elixir of life itself. The journey toward a healthier and happier existence has been illuminated, showcasing how exercise transcends mere movement and nourishes the soul.

Along the way, we navigated common pitfalls, unveiling the mistakes to avoid to ensure a safe and fulfilling exercise regimen. Armed with knowledge and guidance, our seniors have discovered the art of balance, staying in tune with their bodies while cherishing the beauty of progress and rest.

The ink of this book has etched the belief that age is but a number, and with determination and passion, our seniors have rewritten the script of their lives. As we bid farewell to these pages, we celebrate the newfound vigor and the triumphs of our beloved seniors, embracing each day as an opportunity to savor life's joys with unyielding strength.

May "In the Journey of Strength: Empowering Seniors through Fitness" stand as a testament to the unwavering spirit and potential that grace the golden years. Together, we embark on a legacy of hope and health, inspiring generations to come, and empowering seniors to create a legacy that is etched in the annals of time.

The journey does not end here. As the sun sets on this book, a new dawn arises for our seniors, illuminating paths yet to be explored, challenges yet to be conquered, and triumphs yet to be celebrated. In the symphony of life, they have found their rhythm, and with every step, they resound the melody of strength.

As the final chapter draws to a close, let us remember that the journey of strength knows no final destination. Instead, it is an ever-evolving tale of resilience, self-discovery, and boundless potential. Our seniors have found their purpose and passion in the embrace of exercise, and their legacy shall forever inspire us to reach for the stars and embrace our full potential at any age.

So, dear reader, let this book be a reminder that within each of us lies a story of strength, waiting to be awakened.

As we bid adieu to these words, let us continue to seek the beauty of life's journey, with each step bringing us closer to the timeless symphony of strength. The world awaits our legacy, and together, we shall author a tale of hope, love, and limitless possibilities.

With gratitude for every chapter shared, **"6 MINUTES FITNESS AT 5O: CORE EXERCISES FOR BALANCE AND STRENGTH "** celebrates a legacy of empowerment, where the heart of each senior's story intertwines with the vibrant pulse of life's tapestry. Here's to the beauty of the journey and the strength within us all.

THANK YOU!